Diversity, Equity, and Inclusion
Prison the Entry Level Program?
The Long View, Your 42nd Consultation
William R. Yee M.D., J.D.,
Copyright Applied for Sept. 19th, 2023.
ISBN 978-1-304-81148-6

Diversity, Equity, and Inclusion
Prologue

Diversity, Equity, and Inclusion have been hijacked by psychopaths to disrupt culture and raid the treasury.

Diversity, Equity, and Inclusion have been hijacked by psychopaths to censor political discourse necessary to allow different opinions to meet and find mutual values and compromise necessary to allow differences of opinion to coexist peacefully.

Diversity, Equity, and Inclusion is not concerned with the welfare of the educated, rich, and successful. Very often Diversity, Equity, and Inclusion wants to tax the educated, rich, and successful into poverty to fund programs that cannot succeed.

Diversity, Equity, and Inclusion is concerned about the poor who need assistance to achieve the basic needs of life and opportunities to climb the social ladder.

Psychopaths often seize Diversity, Equity, and Inclusion with the object of destroying the social ladder and reducing the United States to a Third World Country with Universal Poverty and a Wealthy Political Aristocracy.

I refer the reader to Thomas Sowell, American economist, and author, for a deeper dive into these topics. He is Black and presents these issues through the lens of a Black, educated, rational, and respected perspective.

My personal experience starts with a Chinese immigrant father and a third-generation Swedish mother.

My mother grew up on a farm in the upper peninsula of Michigan, "Strangely enough, early editions of Webster's Dictionary include a definition of hillbilly as "a Michigan Farmer," May 24, 2022."

I was born in 1947 when "mixed marriages," were not acceptable.

I refer the reader to:
Study finds bias, disgust toward mixed-race couples
Deborah Bach
News and Information
August 17, 2016
https://www.washington.edu/news/2016/08/17/study-finds-bias-disgust-toward-mixed-race-couples/

I grew up in poverty and witnessed my parents' hardships.

I personally have lived Diversity, Equity, and Exclusion in its blatant and subtle forms over the years.

I have overcome many obstacles with hard work and kindness.

I have chosen to work with the lowest tier of social classes in the United States.

Since 1972 I have worked in State Psychiatric Hospitals and Prisons.

"According to data analyzed by the Pew Center on the States, as of Jan. 1, 2008, more than

1. 1 in every 100 adults is behind bars.
2. incarceration is heavily concentrated among men,
3. racial and ethnic minorities, and
4. 20-and 30-year-olds.
5. among men
6. the highest rate
    is with black males aged 20–34.
7. Among women
8. the highest rate
    is black females aged 35–39.

I rely on:
U.S. Incarceration Rates by Race and Sex
National Institute of Justice
https://www.washington.edu/news/2016/08/1
7/study-finds-bias-disgust-toward-mixed-
race-couples/

Average IQ for prison inmates
1. serving sentences of 2 years to life
    is 90.53.

Average IQ for "state jail" inmates
1. serving sentences of 6 months to 2 years
    is 91.15.

I rely on:

Average IQ of prison inmates [Best Guide]
28 November 2021 by personality-test
https://personalityanalysistest.com/average-iq/average-iq-of-prison-inmates-best-guide/

ADHD is overrepresented in prison populations.

"Conclusions
Compared with published general population prevalence,
1. there is a fivefold increase in prevalence of ADHD in youth prison populations (30.1%)
2. and a 10-fold increase in adult prison populations (26.2%)."

I rely on:
A meta-analysis of the prevalence of attention deficit hyperactivity disorder in incarcerated populations.
Young S, Moss D, Sedgwick O, Fridman M, Hodgkins P.
Psychol Med. 2015 Jan;45(2):247-58. doi: 10.1017/S0033291714000762.

Epub 2014 Apr 7. PMID: 25066071; PMCID: PMC4301200

Mental Illness is overrepresented in Prison Populations.

The general population rate for
1. Primary Psychiatric disorder
   from 1.5 to 3.5% of the population
2. Depression is
   5% of adults
   4% among men and 6% among women,
3. alcohol use disorder is 8.6%
4. drug use disorder is
   16.5 percent of the population

In this population, the estimated pooled 1-year prevalence rates,
1. for psychosis were 6·2% (95% CI 4·0–8·6),
2. for major depression, 16·0% (11·7–20·8)
3. for alcohol use disorders, 3·8% (1·2–7·6)
4. for drug use disorders 5·1% (2·9–7·8) f

I rely on:
Severe mental illness and substance use disorders in prisoners in low-income and middle-income countries: a systematic review and meta-analysis of prevalence studies
Gergő Baranyi, MPH
Carolin Scholl, MSc

Seena Fazel, FRCPsych
Vikram Patel, PhD
Stefan Priebe, FRCPsych
Adrian P Mundt, PhD
Open Access Published: April 2019
DOI: https://doi.org/10.1016/S2214-
109X(18)30539-4.

"A troubled past and leaked plans are
common to those who take part in mass
shootings. Most use handguns, NIJ-
supported research shows."

" The Violence Project database spans more
than 50 years, yet 20% of the 167 mass
shootings in that period occurred in the last
five years."

"The most common mass shootings are
1. in workplaces (28.1%),
2. restaurants/bars/nightclubs (14%),
3. retail establishments (12.9%),
4. houses of worship (6.4%),
5. Kindergarten-12th grade elementary,
   middle, and high schools (7.6%),
6. colleges/universities (5.3%),
7. government buildings/places of civic
   importance (2.9%).
8. 22.8% are in other public spaces, like
   neighborhoods and campsites."

Mass Shooter Demographics

1. 97.7% of the perpetrators (N=172) were male,
2. here were four female perpetrators,
3. ages ranged from 11 to 70 years old with a mean of 34.1 (sd=12.2).
4. 52.3% White,
5. 20.9% Black,
6. 8.1% Latinx,
7. 6.4% Asian,
8. 4.2% Middle Eastern, and
9. 1.8% Native American.

The most common location of mass shooting was
1. a workplace (30.8%),
2. retail establishment (16.9%),
3. bar or restaurant (13.4%),
4. residential location (8.1%),
5. outdoors (8.1%),
6. K-12 school (7.6%),
7. place of worship (6.4%),
8. college or university (5.2%), and
9. government or place of civic importance (3.5%).

1. Most perpetrators had a prior criminal record (64.5%) and
2. history of violence (62.8%),
3. including domestic violence (27.9%), and
4. 28.5% had a military history.

The majority of perpetrators
1. died on scene, either by their own hand (38.4%) or t
2. they were killed by law enforcement (20.3%).

Trauma, Suicidality, and Crisis.
The life histories of mass shooters are complex.
1. 31% of them were coded as experiencing severe childhood trauma
2. in K-12 school shooters that number was 68%
3. over 80% of mass shooters were in crisis,
4. their current situation was overwhelming their ability to cope,
5. marked change in behavior prior to their crime,
6. Mass shooters often commit suicide after their attacks,
7. or provoked law enforcement to do it "Suicide-by-Cop"
8. suicide and homicide are linked.
9. 30% of mass shooters were suicidal prior

to the shooting,
10. 39% of mass shooters were suicidal during the shooting.
11. K-12 school shooters 92% were suicidal during the shooting.
12. college/university shooters 100% were suicidal during the shooting.

Mental Illness among mass shooter perpetrators:
1. 19.8% had a history of previous hospitalization for psychiatric reasons,
2. 29.1% had a history of counseling, and
3. 23.3% had a known history of taking psychiatric medication
4. comparable to rates among the U.S. general population; Moore & Mattison, 2017,
5. 15.7% showed evidence of a mood disorder diagnosis,
6. 6.4% showed evidence of an autism spectrum disorder diagnosis,
7. 26.7% showed evidence of a psychotic disorder diagnosis
8. compared to 1% of the general population.
9. The data indicate that symptoms of psychosis
10. played no motivating role in 69% of cases,
11. a small role in 11% of cases,

12. a significant role in 8.7% of cases,
13. psychosis played a primary role in another 10.5% of cases.
14. combining counseling, psychiatric medication, and previous diagnosis 58.7% of perpetrators had a mental health history,
15. somewhat higher than general population levels
    Kessler, Bergulund & Demler, 2005

Motivation Over Time.
1. statistically significant is the fall in shootings motivated by employment issues "Going Postal."

Warning Signs.
1. 48% of all mass shooters leaked their plans, to
2. family members,
2. friends, and
3. colleagues,
4. strangers
5. law enforcement professional
6. face-to-face,
7. over the telephone,
8. in writing, and
9. via the internet and
10. social media.
11. 23.4% of mass shooters left behind a

legacy token
12. such as a "manifesto" that was a clue to their actions.
13. One in five mass shooters (21.6%) studied other mass shooters.
14. 70% of mass shooters knew at least some of their victims
15. K-12 school and workplace shooters were "insiders."
16. current or former students and employees
17. which has implications for physical security measures and
18. the use of active shooter drills in these setting

Firearms.
1. 77.2% of mass shooters use handguns
2. 25.1% use assault rifles
3. 48% use one gun,
4. 22% use two,
5. 15% use 3, and
6. 15% use four or more guns.
7. 32.5% of cases could not be corroborated),
8. 77% of mass shooters purchase at least some of their guns legally,
9. 13% made illegal purchases,
10. 19% stole their guns.
11. Among K-12 school shooters, over 80%

stole their guns from family members
12. background checks may have prevented at least 16 mass shootings,
13. saving over 100 lives,
14. "default proceed" option on federal checks that take longer than three days
15. may have averted the 2015 Charleston church shooting.

Trauma.
1. First, all five of our perpetrator case studies
2. shared Adverse Childhood Experiences.
3. The early lives of our interviewees were punctuated by
4. exposure to physical and sexual abuse,
5. emotional or physical neglect,
6. domestic violence;
7. the death (often suicide) of a parent or
8. experiencing parental separation or divorce.
9. substance use and abuse and
10. bullying.

Research shows that
1. those who have experienced trauma as children
2. were more likely to face a host of difficulties as adults, including
3. having violent relationships,
4. becoming dependent on drugs or alcohol,

5. having a psychiatric disorder and
6. becoming depressed

Beyond the early exposure to violence,
1. all our interviewees developed significant mental health concerns
2. in adolescence, including
3. depression,
4. anxiety,
5. hallucinations and
6. delusions,
7. self-harm, and
8. suicidal ideation.

These mental health concerns
1. cannot be connected
2. in any causal way
3. to the mass shootings that followed,
4. but they were a common,
5. consistent, theme in the data.
6. Further, the participants in this study
7. all reached an identifiable crisis point
8. in the weeks/months before the shooting.

I rely on:
Public Mass Shootings: Database Amasses Details of a Half Century of U.S. Mass Shootings with Firearms, Generating Psychosocial Histories
National Institute of Justice:
NIJ is the research, development and

evaluation agency of the U.S. Department of Justice.
https://nij.ojp.gov/topics/articles/public-mass-shootings-database-amasses-details-half-century-us-mass-shootings
and:
(NEW) Mass Shooting Study What YOU Need to Know
Tom Grieve
212K subscriber
https://www.youtube.com/watch?v=NxW1Mn JgBvs

The purpose of exploring the mental health of the mass shooter was to identify the extent mass shooters overlap with the diversity, equity, and inclusion population. There is a significant overlap.

Now let us expand the scope to identify the diversity, equity, and inclusion population among serial killers, and special cases such as Helen Keller, and feral children.

Feral children do not have any culture to identify with.

We analyzed all published reports of individuals not exposed to syntactic language until puberty:
1. two feral children, who grew up without

hearing any language, and
2. eight deaf linguistic isolates,
3. who grew up communicating to their families using home sign or kitchen sign,
4. a system of gestures which allows them to communicate simple commands,
5. but lacks much in the way of syntax.
6. A common observation in these individuals is
7. the lifelong difficulty understanding syntax and spatial prepositions,
8. even after many years of rehabilitation.
9. This debilitating condition stands in stark contrast to linguistic isolates'
10. performance on memory as well
11. as semantic tests:
12. they could easily remember hundreds of newly learned words
13. and identify previously seen objects by name.
14. The lack of syntactic language comprehension
15. in linguistic isolates
16. may stem from inability to understand words and/or grammar or
17. inability to mentally synthesize known objects
18. into novel configurations.
19. We have previously shown that purposeful construction of novel mental images 20. is the function of the lateral

prefrontal cortex (LPFC)
21. ability to dynamically control posterior cortex neurons.
22. showed decreasing scores in tests that involved greater recruitment
23. of the posterior cortex by the LPFC, and
24. failed in tests that involved greatest recruitment
25. of posterior cortex necessary for mental synthesis of multiple objects.

I rely on:
Linguistically deprived children: meta-analysis of published research underlines the importance of early syntactic language use for normal brain development
Andrey Vyshedskiy, Mahapatra Shreyas, Rita Dunn
doi: https://doi.org/10.1101/166538
Now published in Research Ideas and Outcomes doi: 10.3897/rio.3.e20696

Helen Keller is an example of what all day every day one to one socialization can do for this population.

Anne Sullivan Macy was an American teacher best known for being the instructor and lifelong companion of Helen Keller.

1. On March 3, 1887,
2. Anne Sullivan began teaching six-year
   -old Helen Keller,
3. who lost her sight and hearing,
4. after a severe illness
   at the age of 19 months,
5. Anne Sullivan
6. pioneering "touch teaching"
7. Helen Keller was able to learn to speak
8. read
9. acquire social skills,
10. and graduate from college.
11. Anne Sullivan remained Keller's
    interpreter and constant companion,
12. until the Helen Keller 's death in 1936.

I rely on:
This Day in History
1887
Helen Keller meets Anne Sullivan, her
teacher and 'miracle worker'
History.com Editors
Website NameHISTORY
URLhttps://www.history.com/this-day-in-
history/helen-keller-meets-her-miracle-
worker
Date Accessed November 12, 2023
Publisher A&E Television Networks
Last Updated March 29, 2023
Original Published Date November 24, 2009
https://www.history.com/this-day-in-

history/helen-keller-meets-her-miracle-worker
Now let us look at Serial Killers Ted Bundy and Jeffrey Dahmer.

Jeffrey Lionel Dahmer (/ˈdɑːmər/; May 21, 1960 – November 28, 1994),
1. also known as the Milwaukee Cannibal
2. or the Milwaukee Monster,
3. was an American serial killer and
4. sex offender
5. who killed and
6. dismembered
7. seventeen males
8. between 1978 and 1991.

Although he was
1. diagnosed with
2. borderline personality disorder (BPD),
3. schizotypal personality disorder (StPD),
4. a psychotic disorder,
5. Dahmer was found to be legally sane at his trial.
6. He was convicted of
7. fifteen of the sixteen homicides
8. he had committed in Wisconsin and
9. was sentenced to
10. fifteen terms of life imprisonment on February 17, 1992.
11. Dahmer was later sentenced to a sixteenth term of life imprisonment

12. for an additional homicide committed in Ohio in 1978.
13. November 28, 1994,
14. Dahmer was beaten to death
15. by Christopher Scarver,
16. a fellow inmate at the Columbia Correctional Institution in Portage, Wisconsin after refusing protective segregation.

Childhood
Jeffrey Dahmer
1. was born on May 21, 1960,
2. in Milwaukee, Wisconsin,
3. the first of two sons
4. to Lionel Herbert Dahmer, a Marquette University chemistry student and
5. later a research chemist, and
6. Joyce Annette Dahmer (née Flint),
7. a teletype machine instructor.
8. Lionel is of German and Welsh ancestry,
9. Joyce was of English, Norwegian, and Irish ancestry.

Some sources report
1. Dahmer was deprived of attention as an infant.
2. Other sources, however, suggest that Dahmer was generally doted upon
3. as an infant
4. and toddler

5. by both parents,
6. although his mother was known to
   A. be tense,
   B. greedy for both attention and pity,
   C. argumentative with her husband
   C. and their neighbors.

As Dahmer
1. entered first grade,
2. Lionel's studies kept him away from home much of the time.
3. When he was home,
4. his wife a hypochondriac
5. who suffered from depression
6. demanded constant attention and
7. spent an increasing amount of time in bed.
8. On one occasion, she attempted suicide
9. using Equanil.
10. Consequently,
11. neither parent devoted much time to their son,
12. who later recollected that,
13. from an early age,
14. he felt "unsure of the solidity of the Family,"
15. recalling extreme tension and
16. numerous arguments
17. between his parents during his early years.

Dahmer
1. had been an "energetic and happy child"
2. but became notably subdued after double hernia surgery
3. shortly before his fourth birthday,
4. at elementary school,
5. Dahmer was regarded as quiet and timid;
6. one teacher recollected she detected early signs of abandonment
7. due to his father's absence and mother's illnesses,
8. the symptoms of which increased
9. when she became pregnant
10. with her second child.
11. In elementary school,
12. Dahmer had a small number of friends.

In October 1966,
1. the family moved to Doylestown, Ohio.
2. When Joyce gave birth in December,
3. Dahmer was allowed to choose the name of his new baby brother;
4. he chose the name David.
5. The same year,
6. Lionel earned his degree
7. and started work as an analytical chemist in nearby Akron, Ohio.

From an early age,
1. Dahmer manifested an interest in dead animals.
2. His fascination with dead animals may have begun when, at the age of four,
3. he saw his father removing animal bones from beneath the family home.
4. According to Lionel, Dahmer was "oddly thrilled"
5. by the sound the bones made, and
6. became preoccupied with animal bones,
7. which he initially called his "fiddlesticks".
8. He occasionally searched beneath and around the family home
9. for additional bones, and
10. explored the bodies of live animals
11. to discover where their bones were located.

In May 1968, the family moved to Bath Township, Summit County, Ohio. This address was their third in two years, and Dahmer's sixth address since marriage. The home stood in one and a half acres of woodland, with a small hut only a short walk from the house where Dahmer began collecting large insects and the skeletons of small animals, such as chipmunks and squirrels.[32] Some of these remains were preserved in jars of formaldehyde and stowed within the hut.

Two years later,
1. during a chicken dinner,
2. Dahmer asked Lionel
3. what would happen if the chicken bones were placed in bleach.
4. Lionel, pleased by what he believed to be his son's scientific curiosity,
5. demonstrated how to safely bleach and preserve animal bones.
6. Dahmer incorporated these preserving techniques
7. into his bone collecting.
8. He also began collecting dead animals
9. including roadkill
10. which he would dissect and
11. bury beside the hut,
12. with the skulls occasionally placed atop makeshift crosses.

According to one friend,
1. Dahmer explained to him that
2. he was curious as to how animals "fit together".
3. in one instance in 1975,
4. Dahmer decapitated the carcass
5. of a dog before nailing the body to a tree and
6. impaling the skull upon a stick

7. in the woodland behind his house.
8. As a "prank",
9. he later invited a friend to view the display,
10. claiming he had discovered the remains by chance.
11. The same year Lionel taught his son how to preserve animal bones,
12. Joyce began increasing her daily consumption of
    A. Equanil,
    B. laxatives and
    C. sleeping pills,
13. further minimizing her tangible contact
14. with her husband and children.

Adolescence and high school:
1. From his freshman year at Revere High School,
2. Dahmer was seen as an outcast.
3. By age 14,
4. he had begun drinking beer and
5. hard alcohol in the daylight hours,
6. frequently concealing his liquor
7. inside the jacket he wore to school.
8. Dahmer mentioned to one classmate
9. who inquired why he was drinking Scotch
10. in a morning history class
11. that the alcohol he consumed was "my

medicine".
"now labeled as self-medicating?"
12. Although largely uncommunicative,
13. in his freshman year
14. Dahmer was seen by staff as polite and
15. highly intelligent
16. but with average grades.
17. He was a competitive tennis player,
18. and played briefly in the high school band.

When he reached puberty,
1. Dahmer discovered he was gay;
2. he did not tell his parents.
3. In his early teens,
4. he had a brief relationship with another teenage boy,
5. although they never had intercourse.
6. By Dahmer's admission,
7. he began fantasizing about dominating and controlling
8. a completely submissive male partner in his early to mid-teens,
9. and his masturbatory fantasies
10. gradually evolved to his focusing on chests and torsos.
11. These fantasies gradually became intertwined with dissection.
12. When he was about 16,
13. Dahmer conceived a fantasy
14. of rendering unconscious

15. a particular male jogger he found attractive,
16. and then making sexual use of his body.
17. On one occasion, D
18. Dahmer concealed himself in bushes
19. with a baseball bat
20. to lie in wait for this man.
21. However, the jogger
22. did not pass by on that day.
23. Dahmer later admitted
24. this was his first attempt to attack and
25. render an individual submissive to him.

Dahmer
1. was seen by his high school peers
2. as a class clown
3. who often staged pranks,
4. which became known as
5. "Doing a Dahmer";
6. these included bleating and s
7. emulating epileptic seizures
8. or cerebral palsy
9. at school and local stores.
10. Occasionally, Dahmer
11. would perform these antics f
12. or money to purchase alcohol.

By 1977,
1. Dahmer's grades had declined.
2. His parents hired a private tutor,

3. with limited success.
4. The same year, in an attempt to save
   their marriage,
5. his parents attended counseling
   sessions.
6. They continued to quarrel frequently.
7. When Lionel discovered Joyce had
8. engaged in a brief affair in September
   1977,
9. they decided to divorce,
10. telling their sons they wished to do so
    amicably.
11. The process of their divorce
12. soon became increasingly bitter and
    acrimonious,
13. and Lionel moved out of the house
14. in early 1978, at age 18,
15. temporarily residing in a motel
16. on North Cleveland Massillon Road.

In May 1978,
1. Dahmer graduated from high school.
2. A few weeks before his graduation,
3. one of his teachers observed Dahmer
4. sitting close to the school parking lot,
5. drinking several cans of beer.
6. When the teacher threatened to report
   the matter,
7. Dahmer informed him
8. he was experiencing "a lot of problems"
9. at home and that

10. the school's guidance counselor was aware of them.
11. That spring, Joyce–contrary to a court order
12. and without informing Lionel–
13. moved out of the family home
14. with David to live with relatives
15. in Chippewa Falls, Wisconsin.
16. Dahmer had just turned 18 and
17. remained in the family home.
18. Dahmer's parents' divorce was
19. finalized on July 24, 1978.
20. Joyce was awarded custody of
21. her younger son and alimony payments.

I rely on:
Wikipedia
This page was last edited on 12 November 2023, at 18:35 (UTC).
Text is available under the Creative Commons Attribution-ShareAlike License 4.0; additional terms may apply. By using this site, you agree to the Terms of Use and Privacy Policy. Wikipedia® is a registered trademark of the Wikimedia Foundation, Inc., a non-profit organization.

Ted Bundy From Wikipedia, the free encyclopedia
For the 2002 biographical film, see Ted Bundy (film).

Born: Theodore Robert Cowell
November 24, 1946
Burlington, Vermont, U.S.
Died January 24, 1989 (aged 42)
Florida State Prison, Raiford, Florida, U.S.
Cause of death: Execution by electrocution.

Education: Woodrow Wilson High School
Alma mater
University of Washington (BA)

Spouse: Carole Ann Boone
(m. 1980; div. 1986) Children 1

Motive
Possession-Control

Conviction(s)
First-degree murder (x3)
Attempted first-degree murder (x3)
Aggravated kidnapping
Burglary

Criminal penalty
Two death sentences (1979, 1980)
1 to 15 years in prison (1976)

Escaped: June 7, 1977 – June 13, 1977
December 30, 1977 – February 15, 1978

Details
Victims20 confirmed
30 confessed
36+ suspected
Span of crimes1974 – 1978 (Confirmed)
Country: United States
committed in:
California
Colorado
Florida
Idaho
Oregon
Utah
Washington

Date apprehended August 16, 1975

Theodore Robert Bundy (né Cowell;
November 24, 1946 – January 24,
1989) was an American serial killer who
kidnapped, raped and murdered
dozens of young women and girls during
the 1970s and possibly earlier.

After more than a decade of denials, he confessed to 30 murders committed in seven states between 1974 and 1978. His true victim total is unknown.

Bundy often employed charm to disguise his murderous intent when kidnapping victims and extended this tactic vis-a-vis law enforcement, the media, and the criminal justice system to maintain his claims of innocence.

His usual technique involved approaching a female in public and luring her to a vehicle parked in a more secluded area, at which point she would be beaten unconscious, restrained with handcuffs and taken elsewhere to be sexually assaulted and killed.

To this end, Bundy typically simulated having a physical impairment such as an injury to convince his target that he needed assistance with something or would dupe her into believing he was an authority figure.

He frequently revisited the bodies of those he abducted, grooming, and performing sex acts on the corpses until decomposition and destruction by wild animals made further interactions impossible.

He decapitated at least 12 of his victims, keeping their severed heads as mementos in his apartment. On a few occasions, he broke into homes at night and bludgeoned, maimed, strangled and/or sexually assaulted his victims in their sleep.

In 1975, Bundy was arrested and jailed in Utah for aggravated kidnapping and attempted criminal assault. He then became a suspect in a progressively longer list of unsolved homicides in several states.

Facing murder charges in Colorado, Bundy engineered two dramatic escapes and committed further assaults in Florida, including three murders, before his ultimate recapture in 1978.

For the Florida homicides, he received three death sentences, and was executed at Florida State Prison on January 24, 1989.

Biographer Ann Rule characterized him as "a sadistic sociopath who took pleasure from another human's pain and the control he had over his victims, to the point of death and even after."

Bundy once described himself as "the most cold-hearted son of a bitch you'll ever meet", a statement with which attorney Polly Nelson, a member of his last defense team, agreed. "Ted", she wrote, "was the very definition of heartless evil."

Early life

Childhood
Ted Bundy was born Theodore Robert Cowell on November 24, 1946, to Eleanor Louise Cowell (September 21, 1924 – December 23, 2012, known by her middle name).

Ted Bundy was born at the Elizabeth Lund Home for Unwed Mothers, in Burlington, Vermont.
His biological father's identity has never been confirmed.

His original birth certificate apparently assigns paternity to a salesman and United States Air Force veteran named Lloyd Marshall, though a copy of it listed his father as unknown.

Louise claimed she met a war veteran named Jack Worthington, who abandoned her soon after she became pregnant.

Census records reveal that several men by the name of John Worthington and Lloyd Marshall lived near Louise when Bundy was conceived.

Some family members expressed suspicions that Bundy was sired by Louise's own father.

However, in the 2020 documentary film Crazy, Not Insane, psychiatrist Dorothy Otnow Lewis claimed she received a sample of Bundy's blood and that a DNA test had confirmed that Bundy was not the product of incest.

For the first three years of his life, Bundy lived in the Philadelphia neighborhood Roxborough, Pennsylvania, with his maternal grandparents,

Samuel Knecht Cowell (September 23, 1898 – December 4, 1983) and Eleanor Miriam Longstreet (February 16, 1895 – April 25, 1971) who raised him as their son to avoid the social stigma that accompanied birth outside of wedlock at that time.

Family, friends, and even young Ted were told that his grandparents were his parents and that his mother was his older sister.

Bundy eventually discovered the truth, although his recollections of the circumstances varied; he told a girlfriend that a cousin showed him a copy of his birth certificate after calling him a "bastard," but he told biographers Stephen Michaud and Hugh Aynesworth that he had found the certificate himself.

Biographer and true crime writer Ann Rule, who knew Bundy personally, wrote that he did not find out until 1969, when he located his original birth record in Vermont.

Bundy expressed a lifelong resentment toward his mother for never telling him about his real father, and for leaving him to discover his true parentage for himself.

Bundy occasionally exhibited disturbing behavior at an early age.

Louise's younger sister, Julia Cowell, recalled awakening from a nap to find herself surrounded by knives from the kitchen, and her 3-year-old nephew standing by the bed, smiling.

In some interviews, Bundy spoke warmly of his grandparents and told Rule that he "identified with," "respected," and "clung to" his grandfather.

In 1987, however, he and other family members told attorneys that Samuel was a tyrannical bully who beat his wife and dog, swung neighborhood cats by their tails, and expressed racist and xenophobic attitudes.

In one instance, Samuel reportedly threw Julia down a flight of stairs for oversleeping.

He would sometimes speak aloud to unseen presences, and at least once flew into a violent rage when the question of Bundy's paternity was raised.

Bundy described his grandmother as a timid and obedient woman who periodically underwent electroconvulsive therapy for depression and feared to leave their house toward the end of her life.

These descriptions of Bundy's grandparents have been questioned in more recent investigations.

Some locals remembered Samuel as a "fine man," and expressed bewilderment at the reports of him being violent.

"The characterization that [Sam] was a raging alcoholic and animal abuser was a convenient characterization used to make people justify why Ted was the way he was," said one of Bundy's cousins.

"From my limited exposure to him, nothing could be farther from the truth.

His daughters loved him dearly and had nothing but fond memories of him."

In addition, Louise's sister, Audrey Cowell, stated that their mother could not leave her home because she suffered a stroke due to being overweight and was not mentally ill.

Bundy as a high school senior in 1965

In 1950, Louise changed her surname from Cowell to Nelson and, at the urging of multiple family members, left Philadelphia with Ted to live with cousins Alan and Jane Scott in Tacoma, Washington.

In 1951, Louise met Johnny Culpepper Bundy (April 23, 1921 – May 17, 2007), a hospital cook, at an adult singles night at Tacoma's First Methodist Church.

They married later that year and Johnny formally adopted Ted.

Johnny and Louise conceived four children together, and though Johnny tried to include his adopted son in camping trips and other family activities. Bundy remained distant from him. He would later complain to a girlfriend that Johnny "was not his real father", "wasn't very bright," and "didn't make much money."

Bundy varied his recollections of Tacoma in later years.

To Michaud and Aynesworth, he described roaming his neighborhood, picking through trash barrels in search of pictures of naked women and to attorney and author Polly Nelson he said that he perused detective magazines, and crime novels for stories that involved sexual violence, particularly when the stories were illustrated with pictures of dead or maimed women.

In a letter to Rule, however, he asserted that he "never, ever read fact-detective magazines, and shuddered at the thought that anyone would."

He once told Michaud that he would consume large quantities of alcohol and "canvass the community" late at night in search of undraped windows where he could observe women undressing, or "whatever [else] could be seen."

Psychologist Al Carlisle claimed that Bundy "started fantasizing about women he saw while window peeping or elsewhere [and] mimicking the accents of some politicians he listened to on the radio. In essence, he was fantasizing about being someone else, someone important."

Bundy's childhood Tacoma neighbor Sandi Holt described him as a bully, saying, "He liked to terrify people... He liked to be in charge. He liked to inflict pain and suffering and fear."

She also alleged that Bundy engaged in animal cruelty, saying "He hung one of the stray cats in the neighborhood from one of the clothes lines in the backyard, doused it in lighter fluid and set it on fire and I heard that cat squealing."

Bundy also allegedly used to take younger children in the neighborhood into the woods and terrorize them, she said. "He'd take them out there and strip them down, take their clothes," she said. "You'd hear them screaming for blocks, I mean no matter where we were here, we could hear them screaming."

Holt added, "He had a temper. He liked to scare people. One little girl went over the top of one of Ted's tiger traps and got the whole side of her leg slit open with the sharpened point of the stick that she landed on."

Accounts of Bundy's social life also varied. He told journalists Michaud and Aynesworth that he "chose to be alone" as an adolescent because he was unable to understand interpersonal relationships.

He claimed that he had no natural sense of how to develop friendships. "I didn't know what made people want to be friends," Bundy said. "I didn't know what underlay social interactions." "Some people perceived me as being shy and introverted," he said. "I didn't go to dances. I didn't go on beer drinking outings. I was a pretty, you might call me straight, but not a social outcast in any way."

Classmates from Woodrow Wilson High School, however, told Rule that Bundy was "well known and well liked" there, "a medium-sized fish in a large pond."

Bundy's only significant athletic avocation was downhill skiing, which he pursued enthusiastically with stolen equipment and forged lift tickets.

During high school, he was arrested at least twice on suspicion of burglary and motor vehicle theft.

When he was 18 years old, the details of the incidents were expunged from his record, as is customary in Washington and many other states.

University years
After graduating from high school in 1965, Bundy attended the University of Puget Sound (UPS) for one year before transferring to the University of Washington (UW) to study Chinese.

In 1967, he became romantically involved with a UW classmate, Diane Edwards (identified in Bundy biographies by several pseudonyms, most commonly Stephanie Brooks).

"He saw a woman who was the epitome of his dreams," Rule wrote. "

[Edwards] was like no girl he had ever seen before, and he considered her the most sophisticated, the most beautiful creature possible."

Bundy later described Edwards as, "the only woman I ever really loved."

In early-1968, Bundy dropped out of college and worked a series of minimum-wage jobs.

He also volunteered at the Seattle office of Nelson Rockefeller's presidential campaign and became Arthur Fletcher's driver and bodyguard during Fletcher's campaign for Lieutenant Governor of Washington State.

Edwards graduated in the spring of 1968 and left Washington for San Francisco. Bundy visited her later that year after he earned a scholarship to study Chinese at Stanford University that summer.

In August, Bundy attended the 1968 Republican National Convention in Miami.

Shortly thereafter, Edwards ended their relationship and returned to her family home in California, frustrated by what she described as Bundy's immaturity and lack of ambition.

Psychiatrist Dorothy Otnow Lewis would later pinpoint this crisis as "probably the pivotal time in his development".

Devastated by the breakup, Bundy traveled to Colorado and then farther east, visiting relatives in Arkansas and Philadelphia and enrolling for one semester at Temple University.

It was also at this time in early-1969, Rule believed, that Bundy visited the office of birth records in Burlington and confirmed his true parentage.

Bundy was back in Washington by the fall of 1969, when he met Elizabeth Kloepfer (identified in Bundy literature as Meg Anders, Beth Archer, or Liz Kendall), a single mother from Ogden, Utah, who worked as a secretary at the UW School of Medicine.

Their tumultuous relationship would continue well past his initial incarceration in Utah in 1976.

Bundy became a father figure to Kloepfer's daughter Molly, who was 3 years old when he started dating her mother; he remained in her life until she was aged 10, after he had been arrested.

As an adult, Molly wrote of incidents beginning at age 7 in which Bundy was abusive or sexually inappropriate with her.

Her accounts include Bundy hitting her in the face, knocking her down, putting her at risk of drowning, indecent exposure, and sexual touching disguised as accidents or "games".

In mid-1970, Bundy, now focused and goal-oriented, re-enrolled at UW, this time as a psychology major.

He became an honor student and was well regarded by his professors.

In 1971, he took a job at Seattle's Suicide Hotline Crisis Center. There, he met and worked alongside Ann Rule, a former Seattle police officer and aspiring crime writer who would later write one of the definitive Bundy biographies, The Stranger Beside Me.

Rule saw nothing disturbing in Bundy's personality at the time; she described him as "kind, solicitous, and empathetic."

After graduating from UW in 1972, Bundy joined Governor Daniel J. Evans's re-election campaign.

Posing as a college student, he shadowed Evans' opponent, former governor Albert Rosellini, and recorded his stump speeches for analysis by Evans's team.

Evans appointed Bundy to the Seattle Crime Prevention Advisory Committee.

After Evans was re-elected, Bundy was hired as an assistant to Ross Davis, Chairman of the Washington State Republican Party.

Davis thought well of Bundy and described him as "smart, aggressive ... and a believer in the system."

In early-1973, despite mediocre LSAT scores, Bundy was accepted into the law schools of UPS and the University of Utah on the strength of letters of recommendation from Evans, Davis, and several UW psychology professors.

During a trip to California on Republican Party business in the summer of 1973, Bundy rekindled his relationship with Edwards.

She marveled at his transformation into a serious and dedicated professional who was seemingly on the cusp of a significant legal and political career.

Bundy continued to date Kloepfer as well; neither woman was aware of the other. In the fall of 1973, he matriculated at UPS Law School, and continued courting Edwards, who flew to Seattle several times to stay with him. They discussed marriage, and at one point he introduced her to Davis as his fiancée.

In January 1974, Bundy abruptly broke off
all contact with Edwards; her phone calls
and letters went unreturned. When she
finally reached him by phone a month later,
she demanded to know why he had
unilaterally ended their relationship
without explanation.

In a flat, calm voice, he replied, "Diane, I
have no idea what you mean," and hung up.
She never heard from him again.
Bundy later explained, "I just wanted to
prove to myself that I could have married
her"; but Edwards concluded in retrospect
that "Ted's high-power courtship in the
latter part of 1973 had been deliberately
planned, that he had waited all those years
to be in a position of where he could make
her fall in love with him, so that he could
drop her, reject her, as she had rejected
him."

By then, Bundy had begun skipping classes
at law school. By April, he had stopped
attending entirely, as young women began
to disappear in the Pacific Northwest.

First murders:
There is no consensus as to when or where Bundy began killing women.

He told different stories to different people and refused to divulge the specifics of his earliest crimes, even as he confessed in graphic detail to dozens of later murders in the days preceding his execution.

He told Nelson that he attempted his first kidnapping in 1969 in Ocean City but did not kill anyone until sometime in 1971 in Seattle.

He told psychologist Art Norman that he killed two women in Atlantic City while visiting family in Philadelphia in 1969.

Bundy hinted to homicide detective Robert D. Keppel that he committed a murder in Seattle in 1972 and another murder in 1973 that involved a hitchhiker near Tumwater, but he refused to elaborate.

Rule and Keppel both believed that he might have started killing as a teenager.

Bundy's earliest documented homicides were committed in 1974, when he was 27 years old.

By his own admission, he had by then mastered the necessary skills – in the era before DNA profiling – to leave minimal incriminating forensic evidence at crime scenes.

When reviewing the lives of Jeffrey Dahmer and Ted Bundy it is obvious that they confabulated according to circumstances of the moment so that their internal biographies cannot be discerned.

They presented different characters to different people at different times and different places.

They present as living a life of Dungeons and Dragons, role playing different characters.

One can only conclude with confidence that their behavior is consistent with Antisocial Personality and extreme examples of Psychopathic Personality Disorder.

How do they fit into Diversity, Equity, and Inclusion?

Diversity, Equity, and Inclusion is not well served by releasing a criminal population into the community without supervision and without monitoring.

Children are diagnosed with oppositional defiant disorder, when the reality is they are accurately diagnosed as antisocial personality disorder. A Red Flag is buried resulting in long criminal careers prior to incarceration. Ponder James Bulgar's death.

Too Young to Murder? James Bulgar?

From Wikipedia, the free encyclopedia
Murder of James Bulger

Perpetrators
Robert Thompson
Jon Venables

Motive Inconclusive
Verdict: Guilty
Convictions: Murder, abduction
Sentence:
Indefinite sentence in juvenile detention
(paroled after 8 years)

James Patrick Bulger
(16 March 1990– 12 February 1993)
was a two-year-old boy from Kirkby,
Merseyside, England, who was abducted,
tortured, and murdered by two 10-year-old
boys,
Robert Thompson (born 23 August 1982)
and Jon Venables (born 13 August 1982),
on 12 February 1993.

Thompson and Venables led Bulger away
from the New Strand Shopping Centre in
Bootle, after his mother had taken her eyes
off him momentarily.

His mutilated body was found on a railway line two and a half miles (four kilometers) away in Walton, Liverpool, two days after his abduction.

Thompson and Venables were charged on 20 February 1993 with abduction and murder.

They were found guilty on 24 November, making them the youngest convicted murderers in modern British history.

They were sentenced to indefinite detention at Her Majesty's pleasure, and remained in custody until a Parole Board decision in June 2001 recommended their release on a lifelong license at age 18.

A prisoner who has served their minimum term becomes eligible for parole. If the Parole Board agrees to release a prisoner who was sentenced to life, he or she is released on a life license, meaning that he or she will remain on parole for the remainder of their natural lives.

Venables was sent to prison in 2010 for breaching the terms of his license, was released on parole again in 2013, and in November 2017 was again sent to prison for having child sexual abuse images on his computer.

The Bulger case has prompted widespread debate about how to handle young offenders when they are sentenced or released from custody.

Murder:
Victim James Bulger:
Closed-circuit television (CCTV) at the New Strand Shopping Centre in Bootle on 12 February 1993 showed Thompson and Venables casually observing children, apparently selecting a target.

The boys were playing truant from their local primary school, which they did regularly.

Throughout the day, Thompson and Venables were seen shoplifting various items, including sweets, batteries, a troll doll, and a can of blue Humbrol modelling paint.

One of the boys later revealed that they were planning to abduct a child, lead him to the busy road alongside the shopping center, and push him into the oncoming traffic.

That same afternoon, James Bulger, from Kirkby, went with his mother, Denise, to the New Strand Shopping Centre. Whilst inside the A.R. Tym's butcher's shop on the lower floor of the center at around 15:40, Denise, who had let go of her son's hand to pay for her shopping, realized that her son was missing.

Thompson and Venables approached James Bulger, took him by the hand, and led him out of the shopping center. The moment was caught on CCTV at15:42.

Thompson and Venables took Bulger to the Leeds and Liverpool Canal, around 1⁄4 mile (400 meters) from the New Strand Shopping Centre, where they dropped him on his head, and he suffered injuries to his face.

The boys joked about pushing Bulger into the canal.

An eyewitness said that when he saw Bulger at the canal, the boy was "crying his eyes out".

The boys went on a 2+1⁄2-mile (4-kilometre) walk across Liverpool; they were seen by

around 38 people, but most bystanders did
nothing to intervene.

Two people challenged Thompson and
Venables, but they either claimed that
Bulger was their brother, or that he was
lost, and that they were taking him to a
police station.

At one point, the boys took Bulger into a pet
shop, from which they were ejected.
Eventually, the boys arrived in Walton.
With Walton Lane Police Station across the
road, they hesitated, then led Bulger up a
steep bank to a railway line near the former
Walton & Anfield railway station, close to
Walton Park Cemetery.

One of the boys threw the blue paint that
they had shoplifted earlier into Bulger's left
eye.

They kicked him, stomped on him, and
threw bricks and stones at him.

They placed batteries in Bulger's mouth
and may have inserted some into his anus,
although none were found there.

Finally, the boys dropped a 10 kg (22 lb.)
railway fishplate on Bulger.

He sustained 10 skull fractures because of the bar striking his head.

Pathologist Alan Williams said that Bulger suffered so many injuries - 42 in total - that none could be identified as the fatal blow.

Thompson and Venables laid James Bulger across the railway tracks and weighted his head down with rubble, hoping that a train would hit him, and his death would be ruled an accident.

After they left the scene, his body was cut in half by a train.

Bulger's severed body was discovered by a group of children two days later. A forensic pathologist testified that Bulger died before he was struck by the train.

Police suspected that the boys had sexually assaulted Bulger, as his shoes, socks, trousers, and underpants had been removed.

The pathologist's report, which was read out in court, found that Bulger's foreskin had been forcibly pulled back.

When Thompson and Venables were questioned about this aspect of the attack by detectives and a child psychiatrist, Eileen Vizard, the pair were reluctant to give details.

When Venables was let out on parole, his psychiatrist, Susan Bailey, reported that "visiting and revisiting the issue with Jon as a child, and now as an adolescent, he gives no account of any sexual element to the offence."

The police quickly found low-resolution video images of Bulger's abduction from the New Strand Shopping Centre by two unidentified boys.

The railway embankment upon which his body had been discovered was soon adorned with hundreds of bunches of flowers.

The family of one boy, who was detained for questioning but subsequently released, had to flee the city due to threats from vigilantes.

The breakthrough came when a woman, upon seeing slightly enhanced images of the two boys on national television, recognised Venables, and remembered seeing him playing truant with Thompson in the Bootle area that day. She contacted the police, and the boys were arrested.

Legal proceedings:

Arrest:
Mug shots of Venables and Thompson taken at the time of their arrest

The fact that the suspects were so young came as a shock to investigating officers, headed by Detective Superintendent Albert Kirby of Merseyside Police.

Early press reports and police statements had referred to Bulger being seen with "two youths" (suggesting that the killers were teenagers), the ages of the boys being difficult to ascertain from the images captured by CCTV.

Forensic tests confirmed that both boys had the same blue paint on their clothing as found on Bulger's body.

Both had blood on their shoes; the blood on Thompson's shoe was matched to Bulger's through DNA tests.

A pattern of bruising on Bulger's right cheek matched the features of the upper part of a shoe worn by Thompson.

A paint mark in the toecap of one of Venables's shoes indicated he must have used "some force" when he kicked Bulger.

Thompson is said to have asked police whether Bulger had been taken to hospital to "get him alive again."

The boys were each charged with the murder of James Bulger on 20 February 1993, and appeared at South Sefton Youth Court on 22 February 1993, where they were remanded in custody to await trial.

In the aftermath of their arrest, and throughout the media accounts of their trial, the boys were referred to as "Child A" (Thompson) and "Child B" (Venables).

Awaiting trial, they were held in the secure units where they would eventually be sentenced to be detained at Her Majesty's pleasure.

Trial:

Up to 500 protesters gathered at the Magistrates' Court in the Metropolitan Borough of Sefton during the boys' initial court appearances.

The parents of the accused were moved to different parts of the country and assumed new identities following death threats from vigilantes.

The full trial opened at Sessions House, Preston, on 1 November 1993,[9] conducted as an adult trial with the accused in the dock away from their parents, and the judge and court officials in legal regalia.

The boys denied the charges of murder, abduction and attempted abduction.

The attempted abduction charge related to an incident at the New Strand Shopping Centre earlier on 12 February 1993, the day of Bulger's death.

Thompson and Venables had attempted to lead away another two-year-old boy but had been prevented by the boy's mother.

Each boy sat in view of the court on raised chairs so they could see out of the dock designed for adults and were accompanied by two social workers and guards.

Although they were separated from their parents, they were within touching distance when their families attended the trial.

News stories reported the demeanor of the defendants.

These aspects were later criticized by the European Court of Human Rights, which ruled in 1999 that they had not received a fair trial by being tried in public in an adult court.

Thompson and Venables were considered by the court to be capable of "mischievous discretion", meaning an ability to act with criminal intent as they were mature enough to understand that they were doing something seriously wrong.

A child psychiatrist, Eileen Vizard, who interviewed Thompson before the trial, was asked in court whether he would know the difference between right and wrong, that it was wrong to take a young child away from his mother, and that it was wrong to cause injury to a child.

Vizard replied, "If the issue is on the balance of probabilities, I think I can answer with certainty."

Vizard also said that Thompson was suffering from post-traumatic stress disorder after the attack on Bulger.

Susan Bailey, the Home Office's forensic psychiatrist who interviewed Venables, said unequivocally that he knew the difference between right and wrong.

Thompson and Venables did not speak during the trial, and the case against them was based to a large extent on the more than 20 hours of tape-recorded police interviews with the boys, which were played back in court.

Thompson was considered to have taken the leading role in the abduction process, though it was Venables who had apparently initiated the idea of taking Bulger to the railway line.

Venables later described how Bulger seemed to like him, holding his hand and allowing him to pick him up on the meandering journey to the scene of his murder.

Laurence Lee, who was the solicitor of Venables during the trial, later said that Thompson was one of the most frightening children he had seen and compared him to the Pied Piper.

After his appearances in court, Venables would strip off his clothes, saying: "I can smell James like a baby smell."

The prosecution admitted a number of exhibits during the trial, including a box of 27 bricks, a blood-stained stone, Bulger's underpants, and the rusty iron bar described as a railway fishplate.

The pathologist spent 33 minutes outlining the injuries sustained by Bulger; many of those to his legs had been inflicted after he was stripped from the waist down.

Brain damage was extensive and included a hemorrhage.

The boys, by then aged 11, were found guilty of Bulger's murder at the Preston court on 24 November 1993, becoming the youngest convicted murderers of the 20th century.

The judge, Mr Justice Morland, told Thompson and Venables that they had committed a crime of "unparalleled evil and barbarity ... In my judgment, your conduct was both cunning and very wicked."

Morland sentenced them to be detained at Her Majesty's pleasure, with a recommendation that they should be kept in custody for "very, very many years to come", recommending a minimum term of eight years.

At the close of the trial, the judge lifted reporting restrictions and allowed the names of the killers to be released, saying: "I did this because the public interest overrode the interest of the defendants ... There was a need for an informed public debate on crimes committed by young children."

David Omand later criticized this decision and outlined the difficulties created by it in his 2010 review of the probation service's handling of the case.

Post-trial:
Shortly after the trial, and after the judge had recommended a minimum sentence of eight years, Lord Taylor of Gosforth, the Lord Chief Justice, recommended that the two boys should serve a minimum of ten years, which would have made them eligible for release in February 2003 at the age of 20.

The editors of The Sun handed a petition bearing nearly 280,000 signatures to Michael Howard, the Home Secretary, in a bid to increase the time spent by both boys in custody.

This campaign was successful, and Howard announced in July 1994 that the boys would be kept in custody for a minimum of fifteen years, meaning that they would not be considered for release until February 2008, by which time they would be 25 years old.

Lord Donaldson criticized Howard's intervention, describing the increased tariff as "institutionalized vengeance ... [by] a politician playing to the gallery".

The increased minimum term was overturned in 1997 by the House of Lords that ruled it "unlawful" for the Home Secretary to decide on minimum sentences for young offenders.

The High Court of Justice and European Court of Human Rights have since ruled that although the parliament may set minimum and maximum terms for individual categories of crime, it is the responsibility of the trial judge, with the benefit of all the evidence and argument from both prosecution and defense counsel, to determine the minimum term in individual criminal cases.

Tony Blair, then Shadow Home Secretary, gave a speech in Wellingborough during which he said: "We hear of crimes so horrific they provoke anger and disbelief in equal proportions ... These are the ugly manifestations of a society that is becoming unworthy of that name."

Prime Minister John Major said that "society needs to condemn a little more and understand a little less."

The trial judge Mr Justice Morland stated that exposure to violent videos might have encouraged the actions of Thompson and Venables; this was disputed by David Maclean, the Minister of State at the Home Office at the time, who said that police had found no evidence linking the case with "video nasties".

Some British tabloid newspapers claimed that the attack on Bulger was inspired by the film Child's Play 3 and campaigned for the rules on "video nasties" to be tightened.

During the police investigation, it emerged that Child's Play 3 was one of the films that Venables's father had rented in the months prior to the killing, but it was not proven that Venables had ever watched it.

One scene in the film shows the malevolent doll Chucky being splashed with blue paint during a paintball game.

A Merseyside detective said, "We went through something like 200 titles rented by the Venables family.

There were some you or I wouldn't want to see, but nothing - no scene, or plot, or dialogue - where you could put your finger on the freeze button and say that influenced a boy to go out and commit murder."

Inspector Ray Simpson of Merseyside Police commented: "If you are going to link this murder to a film, you might as well link it to The Railway Children." The Criminal Justice and Public Order Act 1994clarified the rules on the availability of certain types of video material to children.[9][56]

Detention:
The Red Bank secure unit in 2022

After the trial, Thompson was held at the Barton Moss Secure Care Centre in Manchester.

Venables was detained in Vardy House, a small eight-bedded unit at Red Bank secure unit in St. Helens on Merseyside.

These locations were not publicly known until after the boys' release.

Details of the boys' lives were recorded twice daily on running sheets and signed by the member of staff who had written them; the records were stored at the units and copied to officials in Whitehall.

The boys were taught to conceal their real names and the crime they had committed which resulted in their being in the units.

Venables' parents regularly visited their son at Red Bank, just as Thompson's mother did, every three days, at Barton Moss.

The boys received education and rehabilitation; despite initial problems, Venables was said to have eventually made good progress at Red Bank, resulting in him being kept there for the full eight years, despite the facility only being a short-stay remand unit.

Both boys were reported to suffer post-traumatic stress disorder, and Venables in particular told of experiencing nightmares and flashbacks of the murder.

Appeal and release:
In 1999, lawyers for Thompson and Venables appealed to the European Court of Human Rights that the boys' trial had not been impartial, since they were too young to follow proceedings and understand an adult court.
The court dismissed their claim that the trial was inhuman and degrading treatment but upheld their claim they were denied a

fair trial by the nature of the court proceedings.

The court also held that the Home Secretary's intervention had led to a "highly charged atmosphere", which resulted in an unfair judgment.

On 15 March 1999, the court in Strasbourg ruled by 14 votes to five that there had been a violation of Article 6 of the European Convention on Human Rights regarding the fairness of the trial of Thompson and Venables, stating: "The public trial process in an adult court must be regarded in the case of an 11-year-old child as a severely intimidating procedure."

In September 1999, Bulger's parents appealed to the European Court of Human Rights but failed to persuade the court that a victim of a crime has the right to be involved in determining the sentence of the perpetrator.

The European Court case led to the new Lord Chief Justice, Lord Woolf, reviewing the minimum sentence.

In October 2000, he recommended the tariff be reduced from ten to eight years, adding that Her Majesty's Young Offender Institution was a "corrosive atmosphere" for the juveniles.

In June 2001, after a six-month review, the parole board ruled the boys were no longer a threat to public safety and could be released, as their minimum tariff had expired in February of that year. Home Secretary David Blunkett approved the decision, and they were released a few weeks later on lifelong license after serving eight years. It was reported that both boys "were given new identities and moved to secret locations under a 'witness protection'-style program."

This was supported by the fabrication of passports, national insurance numbers, qualification certificates, and medical records.

Blunkett added his own conditions to their license and insisted on being sent daily updates on the boys 'actions.

The terms of their release included the following: they were not allowed to contact each other or Bulger's family; they were prohibited from visiting the Merseyside region; curfews may be imposed on them, and they must report to probation officers.

If they breached the rules or were deemed a risk to the public, they could be returned to prison.

An injunction was imposed on the media after the trial, preventing the publication of details about Thompson and Venables.

The worldwide injunction was kept in force following their release on parole, so their new identities and locations could not be published.

In 2001, Blunkett stated: "The injunction was granted because there was a real and strong possibility that their lives would be at risk if their identities became known."

Later events:
In the months after the trial, and following the birth of their second son, the marriage of Bulger's parents, Ralph and Denise, broke down; they divorced in 1995.

Denise married Stuart Fergus, with whom she had two sons.

Ralph also remarried and had three daughters with his second wife.

The Observer revealed that both Venables and Thompson had passed A-Levels during their sentences.

The paper also stated that Bulger family's lawyers had consulted psychiatric experts in order to present the parole panel with a report that suggested that Thompson is an undiagnosed psychopath, citing his lack of remorse during his trial and arrest.

The report was ultimately dismissed; however, his lack of remorse at the time, in stark contrast to Venables, led to considerable scrutiny from the parole panel.

Upon
release, both Thompson and Venables had lost all trace of their Scouse accent.

In a psychiatric report prepared in 2000 before Venables's release, he was described as posing a "trivial" risk to the public and unlikely to reoffend. The chances of his successful rehabilitation were described as "very high".

The Manchester Evening News published details that suggested the names of the secure institutions in which the pair were housed, in breach of the injunction against publicity that had been renewed early in 2001.

In December that year, the paper was fined £30,000 for contempt of court and ordered to pay costs of £120,000.

No significant publication or vigilante action against Thompson or Venables has occurred.

Despite this, Bulger's mother, Denise, told how in 2004 she received a tip-off from an anonymous source that helped her locate Thompson.

Upon seeing him, she was "paralyzed with hatred", and was unable to confront him.

In April 2007, documents released under the Freedom of Information Act 2000 confirmed that the Home Office had spent £13,000 on an injunction to prevent a foreign magazine from revealing the new identities of Thompson and Venables.

On 14 March 2008, an appeal to set up a Red Balloon Learner Centre in Merseyside in memory of James Bulger was launched by his mother and Esther Rantzen.

A memorial garden in Bulger's memory was created in Sacred Heart Primary School in his hometown of Kirkby, the school he would have been expected to attend had he not been murdered.

In March 2010, a call was made by England's Children's commissioner Maggie Atkinson to raise the age of criminal responsibility from ten to twelve.

She said that the killers of James Bulger should have undergone "programs" to help turn their lives around, rather than being prosecuted.

The Ministry of Justice rejected the call, saying that children over the age of ten knew the difference "between bad behavior and serious wrongdoing".

In April 2010, a 19-year-old man from the Isle of Man was given a three-month suspended prison sentence for falsely claiming in a Facebook message that one of his former colleagues was Thompson.

In passing sentence, Deputy High Bailiff Alastair Montgomerie said that the teenager had "put that person at significant risk of serious harm" and in a "perilous position" by making the allegation.

In March 2012, a 26-year-old man from Chorley, Lancashire, was arrested after allegedly setting up a Facebook group with the title "What happened to Jamie Bulger was f**king hilarious." The man's computer was seized for further investigations.

On 25 February 2013, the Attorney General's Office announced that it was instituting contempt of court proceedings against several people who had allegedly published photographs online showing Thompson or Venables as adults.

A spokesman commented: "There are many different images circulating online claiming to be of Venables or Thompson; potentially innocent individuals may be wrongly identified as being one of the two men and placed in danger. The order, and its enforcement, is therefore intended to protect not only Venables and Thompson, but also those members of the public who have been incorrectly identified as being one of the two men."

Images which were claimed to be of Venables and Thompson were posted on Facebook and Twitter. The posts were seen by 24,000 people. According to BBC legal correspondent Clive Coleman, the purpose of the prosecution was to ensure that the public was aware that Internet users were also subject to the law of contempt.

On 27 November 2013, a man from Liverpool received a fourteen-month suspended prison sentence for posting images on Twitter claiming to show Venables.

On 14 July 2016, a woman from Margate in Kent was jailed for three years after sending Twitter messages to Bulger's mother, in which she posed as one of his killers, and as Bulger's ghost.
The sentence was reduced to 2+1⁄2 years on appeal.

On 25 October, a man was jailed for 26 weeks for stalking Denise Fergus; he had previously received a police warning for stalking her in 2008.

On 31 January 2019, a man and a woman pleaded guilty to eight contempt of court offences at the High Court after they admitted to posting photos on social media that they claimed identified Venables; both received suspended prison sentences.

On 13 March 2019, actress Tina Malone was given an eight-month suspended prison sentence for posting Venables's identity on Facebook.

In January 2020, a 53-year-old woman from Ammanford in South Wales received a prison sentence of eight months, suspended for 15 months.

In November 2017, she had published an alleged photograph of Venables on Facebook, with the advice "share this as much as possible".

Lord Justice Nigel Davis said that the offence was "close to the line" for an immediate prison sentence but suspended the sentence, after observing an early admission of guilt and remorse by the woman.

Later life of Jon Venables:
Relationships and other misdemeanors.

Shortly before his 2001 release, when aged 17, Venables was alleged to have had sex with a woman who worked at the Red Bank secure unit where he was held.

In April 2011, in the aftermath of his 2010 imprisonment, these allegations were outlined in a Sunday Times Magazine article written by David James Smith, who had been following the Bulger case since the 1993 trial, and again later in a BBC documentary titled Jon Venables: What Went Wrong?

The female staff member was suspended for sexual misconduct; she never returned to work at Red Bank.

A spokesperson for St Helens Borough Council denied that the incident had been covered up, saying: "All allegations were thoroughly investigated by an independent team on the orders of the Home Office and chaired by Arthur de Frischling, a retired prison governor."

Venables began living independently in March 2002. Sometime thereafter, he began a relationship with a woman who had a five-year-old child; it is not known whether Venables had already begun downloading child abuse images at the time of dating the woman, although he denies having ever met the child.

In 2005, when Venables was 23, his probation officer met another girlfriend of his, who was aged 17.

After a number of "young girlfriends", it was presumed that Venables was having a delayed adolescence.

After a period of apparently reduced supervision, Venables began excessively drinking, taking drugs, and downloading child abuse images, as well as visiting Merseyside, which was a breach of his license.

In 2008, a new probation officer said that he spent "a great deal of leisure time" playing video games and on the Internet.

In September that year, Venables was arrested on suspicion of affray, following a fight outside a nightclub; he claimed he was acting in self-defense, and the charges were later dropped after he agreed to go on an alcohol-awareness course.

Three months later, he was found to be in possession of cocaine; he was subjected to a curfew.

On two occasions, Venables revealed his true identity to a friend.

2010 imprisonment
On 2 March 2010, the Ministry of Justice revealed that Venables had been returned to prison for an unspecified violation of the terms of his license of release.

Justice Secretary Jack Straw said that Venables had been returned to prison because of "extremely serious allegations", and said that he was "unable to give further details of the reasons for Jon Venables's return to custody, because it was not in the public interest to do so".

On 7 March, media reports said that he had been accused of offences related to possession of child sexual abuse material.

In a statement to the House of Commons on 8 March 2010, Straw reiterated that it was "not in the interest of justice" to reveal the reason Venables had been returned to custody.

Baroness Butler-Sloss, the judge who made the decision to grant Venables anonymity in 2001, warned that Venables could be killed if his identity was revealed.

Bulger's mother, Denise Fergus, said she was angry that the parole board did not tell her that Venables had been returned to prison, and called for his anonymity to be removed if he was charged with a crime.

A spokesperson for the Ministry of Justice said that there was a worldwide injunction against publication of either killer's location or new identity.

Venables's return to prison revived a false claim that a man from Fleetwood, Lancashire, was Venables. While the claim was reported and dismissed in September 2005, it reappeared in March 2010 when it was circulated widely via SMS messages and Facebook.

Chief Inspector Tracie O'Gara of Lancashire Constabulary said: "An individual who was targeted four-and-a-half years ago was not Jon Venables, and now he has left the area."

On 21 June 2010, Venables was charged with possession and distribution of indecent images of children.

It was alleged that he had downloaded 57 indecent images of children over a 12-month period to February 2010, and had allowed other people to access the files through a peer-to-peer network.

Venables faced two charges under the Protection of Children Act 1978.

On 23 July, Venables appeared at a court hearing at the Old Bailey via a video link, visible only to the judge hearing the case.

He pleaded guilty to charges of downloading and distributing child sexual abuse material, and was sentenced to two years' imprisonment.

At the court hearing, it emerged that Venables had posed in online chat rooms as 35-year-old Dawn "Dawnie" Smith, a married woman from Liverpool who boasted about abusing her 8-year-old daughter, in the hope of obtaining further child sexual abuse material.

Venables had contacted his probation officer in February 2010, fearing that his new identity had been compromised at his place of work.

When the officer arrived at his flat, Venables was trying to remove or destroy the hard drive of his computer with a knife and a tin opener.

The officer's suspicions were aroused, and the computer was taken away for examination leading to the discovery of the child sexual abuse material, which included children as young as two being raped by adults, and penetrative rape of seven- or eight-year-olds.

The judge, Mr Justice David Bean, ruled that Venables's new identity could not be revealed, but the media were allowed to report that he had been living in Cheshire at the time of his arrest

The High Court also heard that Venables had been arrested on suspicion of affray in September 2008, following a drunken street fight with another man.

Later that year, he was cautioned for possession of cocaine.

In November 2010, a review of the National Probation Service handling of the case by David Omand found that probation officers could not have prevented Venables from downloading child sexual abuse material.

Harry Fletcher, the assistant general secretary of the National Association of Probation Officers, said that only 24-hour surveillance would have stopped Venables.

Venables was eligible for parole in July 2011.

On 27 June 2011, the parole board decided that he would remain in custody, and that his parole would not be considered again for at least another year.

New identity
On 4 May 2011, it was reported that Venables would once again be given a new identity, following what was described as a "serious security breach", which revealed an identity that he had been using before his imprisonment in 2010; details of the breach could not be reported for legal reasons.

A spokesperson for the Ministry of Justice commented: "Such a change of identity is extremely rare, and granted only when the police assess that there is clear and credible evidence of a sustained threat to the offender's life on release into the community."

The incident occurred after a man from Exeter posted photographs on a website devoted to identifying pedophiles, allegedly showing Venables as an adult, and revealing his name.

2013 parole hearing and release:
In November 2011, it was reported that officials had decided that Venables would stay in prison for the foreseeable future, as he would be likely to reveal his true identity if released.

A Ministry of Justice spokesperson declined to comment on the reports.

On 4 July 2013, it was reported that the Parole Board for England and Wales had approved the release of Venables.

On 3 September 2013, it was reported that Venables had been released from prison.
2017 imprisonment

On 23 November 2017, it was reported that Venables had again been recalled to prison for possession of child sexual abuse imagery.

The Ministry of Justice declined to comment on the reports.

On 5 January 2018, Venables was charged with unspecified offences relating to indecent images of children.

On 7 February, Venables pleaded guilty to possession of indecent images of children for a second time.

He pleaded guilty via video link to three charges of making indecent images of children, and one of owning a "pedophile manual", that included advice for would-be child molesters, including instructions on child grooming and evading detection.

He admitted being in possession of 392 category A, 148 category B, and 630 category C child sexual abuse images, and was sentenced to three years and four months in prison.

In September 2020, he was denied parole. His next parole hearing is scheduled to take place in November 2023.

2019 legal challenge to lift anonymity refused:
On 4 March 2019, Bulger's father, Ralph, lost a legal challenge to lift the lifelong order protecting Venables's anonymity. Judge Andrew McFarlane turned down the request, saying that the "uniquely notorious" nature of the case meant there is "a strong possibility, if not a probability, that if his identity were known, he would be pursued, resulting in grave and possibly fatal consequences."

Potential overseas resettlement:
In late June 2019, it was reported that British officials had considered resettling Venables in Canada, Australia, or New Zealand, due to the high costs behind protecting his anonymity.

British authorities had reportedly spent £65,000 in legal fees to keep Venables' identity a secret.

In response to media coverage, Prime Minister Jacinda Ardern remarked that, due to his criminal history, Venables would need an exemption under New Zealand's Immigration Act 2009, and that he should "not bother" applying.

In popular culture:
In August 2001, a stage play titled The Age of Consent by Peter Morris was performed at the Edinburgh Festival Fringe.

The play featured an 18-year-old character called Timmy, who was due to be released from a secure unit after luring a toddler away from his mother and beating him to death.

The play generated controversy due to the similarities between the character and James's killers.

Although she had not seen the play, Denise Fergus denounced it as a work that was "just designed to try and shock people and grab publicity" and that "anyone who would stoop so low as to use my son's death as a subject for comedy is sick and pathetic."

In response to the controversy, Morris stated that the humour in his play was "never at the expense of the various people, Mrs Fergus included, who have suffered so much in the aftermath of James's murder".

He commented that the work "is emphatically not a comedy" but instead "intended as a serious moral examination of what contemporary society is doing to children".

In June 2007, a computer game based on the television series Law & Order, titled Law & Order: Double or Nothing (made in 2003), was withdrawn from stores in the UK following reports that it contained an image of Bulger. The image in question is the CCTV frame of Bulger being led away by Thompson and Venables.

The scene in the game involves a computer-generated detective pointing out the picture, which is meant to represent a fictional child abduction that the player is then asked to investigate.

Bulger's family, along with many others, complained, and the game was subsequently withdrawn by its UK distributor, GSP.

The game's developer, Legacy Interactive, released a statement in which it apologized for the image's inclusion in the game; according to the statement, the image's use was "inadvertent", and took place "without any knowledge of the crime, which occurred in the UK, and was minimally publicized in the United States."

In 2008, Swedish playwright Niklas Rådström used the interview transcripts from interrogations with the murderers and their families to recreate the story.

His play, Monsters, opened to mixed reviews at the Arcola Theatre in London in May 2009.

In August 2009, Australia's Seven Network used real footage of the abduction to promote its crime drama City Homicide.

The use of the footage was criticized by Bulger's mother, and Seven apologized.

On 24 August, co-hosts on Seven's breakfast show Sunrise asked whether the killers were now living in Australia, in an apparent tie-in with that week's episode of City Homicide.

They answered the question the next day, relaying the Australian government's denial that the killers had been settled in the country.

A storyline in Hollyoaks, set to begin in December 2009, was cancelled after the makers gave Bulger's mother Denise Fergus a special screening.

The storyline was to feature Loretta Jones and her friend Chrissy, who had been given new identities before arriving in the village, after being convicted of murdering a child at the age of 12.

The critical theorist Terry Eagleton introduced his 2010 book On Evil with the story of Bulger's murder.

In January 2019, the short film Detainment was nominated for Best Live Action Short Film at the 91st Academy Awards.

The film is based on transcripts of the police interviews with Thompson and Venables after their arrests.

The nomination was criticized by Bulger's mother, who was not consulted before the film's release.

Bulger's mother circulated a petition to have the film removed from the Nominations.

Vincent Lambe, the film's director, said he would not be withdrawing the film, saying that "it would defeat the purpose of making the film".

Penry v. Lynaugh, 492 U.S. 302 (1989)
JUSTICE BRENNAN, with whom JUSTICE MARSHALL joins, concurring in part and dissenting in part.

Mental Retardation Through the Lens of the Death Penalty

JUSTICE BRENNAN, with whom JUSTICE MARSHALL joins, concurring in part and dissenting in part.

1. I agree that the jury instructions given at sentencing in this case deprived petitioner of his constitutional right to have a jury consider all mitigating evidence that he presented before sentencing him to die.

2. I would also hold, however, that the Eighth Amendment prohibits the execution of offenders who are mentally retarded, and who thus lack the full degree of responsibility for their crimes that is a predicate for the constitutional imposition of the death penalty.

I dissented in Teague v. Lane, 489 U. S. 288, 489 U. S. 326 (1989), and

1. I continue to believe that the plurality's unprecedented curtailment of the reach of the Great Writ in that case was without foundation.

2. The Teague plurality adopted for no adequate reason a novel threshold test for federal review of state criminal convictions that, subject to narrow exceptions, precludes federal courts from considering a vast array of important federal questions on collateral review, and thereby both prevents the vindication of personal constitutional rights and deprives our society of a significant safeguard against future violations.

3. In this case, the Court compounds its error by extending Teague's notion that new rules will not generally be announced on collateral review to cases in which a habeas petitioner challenges the constitutionality of a capital sentencing procedure.
4. This extension means that a person may be killed although he or she has a sound constitutional claim that would have

barred his or her execution had this Court only announced the constitutional rule before his or her conviction and sentence became final.

5. It is intolerable that the difference between life and death should turn on such a fortuity of timing, and beyond my comprehension that a majority of this Court will so blithely allow a State to take a human life though the method by which sentence was determined violates our Constitution.

6. I say the Court takes this step "blithely" advisedly.

7. The Court extends Teague
   A. without the benefit of briefing or
   B. oral argument.

8. Teague, indeed, was decided only after we had heard argument in this Case.

9. Rather than postponing decision on the important issue whether Teague should be extended to capital cases until it is presented in a
case in which it may be briefed and argued,

10. the Court rushes to decide Teague's applicability in such circumstances here. It does so in two sentences, ante at 492 U. S. 313-314,

A. saying merely that not to apply Teague

B. would result in delay in killing the prisoner and

C, in a lack of finality.

11. There is not the least hint that the Court has even considered whether different rules might be called for in capital cases,

12. let alone any sign of reasoning justifying the extension.

13. Such peremptory treatment of the issue is facilitated, of course, by the Court's decision to reach the Teague question without allowing counsel to set out the opposing arguments.

14. Though I believe Teague was wrongly decided, and the Court's precipitous decision to extend Teague to capital cases an error, nevertheless,

15. if these mistakes are to be made law,

16. I agree that the Court's discussion of the question whether the jury had an opportunity to consider Penry's mitigating evidence in answering Texas' three "special issues" does not establish a "new rule."

17. I thus join Part II-B of the Court's opinion, and all of Parts I and III.

18. I also agree that there is an exception to Teague so that new rules "prohibiting a certain category of punishment for a class of defendants because of their status or offense" may be announced in, and applied to, cases on collateral review. Ante at 492 U. S. 330.

19. I thus join Part IV-A of the Court's opinion.

II
A majority of the Court today reaffirms, in this case and in Stanford v. Kentucky, post at 492 U. S. 382 (O'CONNOR, J., concurring in part and concurring in judgment); post at 492 U. S. 393 (BRENNAN, J., dissenting), the well-established principle that

1. "application of the death penalty to particular categories of crimes

or classes of offenders violates the Eighth Amendment [if] it"

2. "makes no measurable contribution to acceptable goals of punishment
and hence is nothing more than the purposeless and needless imposition of pain and suffering"

3. "or [if] it is 'grossly out of proportion to the severity of the crime."

4. The contours of these these two inquiries are clear.

5. We gauge whether a punishment is disproportionate by

6. comparing "the gravity of the offense,"
    A. understood to include not only the injury caused,
    B. but also the defendant's moral culpability,

7. with "the harshness of the penalty."

8. In my view, execution of the mentally retarded
    A. is unconstitutional under both these strands of Eighth Amendment analysis.

9. I agree with JUSTICE O'CONNOR

10. that one question to be asked in determining whether the execution of mentally retarded offenders is always unconstitutional because disproportionate

11. is whether the mentally retarded, as a class,

12. "by virtue of their mental retardation alone, . . .

13. inevitably lack
    A. the cognitive,
    B. volitional, and
    C. moral capacity

14. to act with the degree of culpability

15. associated with the death penalty."

16. "Mental retardation" is defined by the American Association on Mental Retardation (AAMR) as

17. "significantly subaverage general intellectual functioning

18. existing concurrently with deficits in adaptive behavior

19. and manifested during the developmental period."

20. To fall within this definition, an individual

21. must be among the approximately two percent of the population

22. with an IQ below 70 on standardized measures of intelligence,

23. and in addition must be subject to

24. "significant limitations in [his or her]

25. effectiveness in meeting the standards of
A. maturation,
B. learning,
C. personal independence,
D. and/or social responsibility
E. that are expected for his or her age level and
F. and cultural group,"

26. Thus, while as between the
A. mildly,
B. moderately,
C. severely, and

D. profoundly mentally retarded,

27. with IQs ranging from 70 to below 20,

28. there are indeed "marked variations in the degree of deficit manifested,"

29. it is also true that "all individuals [designated as mentally retarded]

30. share the common attributes of
   A. low intelligence and
   B. inadequacies in adaptive behavior."

30. In light of this clinical definition of mental retardation,

31. I cannot agree that the undeniable fact that

32. mentally retarded persons have "diverse capacities and life experiences,"

33. is of significance to the Eighth Amendment

34. proportionality analysis we must conduct in this case.

35. "Every individual who has mental retardation" --

36. irrespective of his or her precise
capacities or experiences –
37. has "a substantial disability in
A. cognitive ability and
B. adaptive behavior."

38. This is true even of the "highest
functioning individuals in the mild'
retardation category,"

39. and of course of those like Penry whose
cognitive and behavioral disabilities
place them on the borderline between
mild and moderate retardation.

40. "reduced ability is found in every
dimension of the individual's
functioning,
A. including his language,
B. communication,
C. memory,
D. attention,
E. ability to control impulsivity,
F. moral development,
G. self-concept,
H. self-perception,
J. suggestibility,
K. knowledge of basic information,
L. and general motivation."

41. Though individuals, particularly those
who are mildly retarded,
A. may be quite capable of overcoming
these limitations
B. to the extent of being able to
"maintain themselves independently
C. or semi-independently in the
community,"

42. nevertheless, the mentally retarded
A. by definition "have a reduced ability
to
B. cope with and
C. function in the everyday world."

43. The impairment of a mentally retarded
offender's
A. reasoning abilities,
B. control over impulsive behavior,
C. and moral development,
D. in my view, limits his or her
culpability
E. so that, whatever other punishment
might be appropriate,
F. the ultimate penalty of death
G. is always and necessarily
disproportionate
H. to his or her blameworthiness,
I. and hence is unconstitutional.

44. Even if mental retardation alone were

   A. not invariably associated with a lack
      of the degree of culpability
   B. upon which death as a proportionate
      punishment is predicated,

45. I would still hold the execution of
The mentally retarded to be
unconstitutional.

46. If there are among the mentally
retarded exceptional individuals as
responsible for their actions as persons
who suffer no such disability

47. the individualized consideration
afforded at sentencing fails to ensure
that they are the only mentally retarded
offenders who will be picked out to
receive a death sentence.

48. The consideration of mental
retardation

49. as a mitigating factor is inadequate

50. to guarantee, as the Constitution
requires,

51. that an individual who is not fully
blameworthy for his or her crime

52. because of a mental disability

53. does not receive the death penalty.

54. That "sentencers

55. can consider and give effect to mitigating evidence

56. of mental retardation

57. in imposing sentence"

58. provides no assurance

59. that an adequate individualized determination

60. of whether the death penalty is a proportionate punishment

61. will be made

62. at the conclusion of each capital trial.

63. At sentencing, the judge

64. or jury

65. considers an offender's level of blameworthiness

66. only along with a host of other factors

67. that the sentencer may decide
    outweigh

68. any want of responsibility.

69. The sentencer is free

70. to weigh a mentally retarded offender's
    relative lack of culpability

71. against the heinousness of the crime

72. and other aggravating factors, and

73. to decide that even the most retarded
    and irresponsible of offenders

74. should die.

75. Indeed, a sentencer will entirely
    discount an offender's retardation

76. as a factor mitigating against
    imposition of a death sentence

77. if it adopts this line of reasoning:

78: "It appears to us that there is all the
   more reason to execute a killer if he is
   also . . .
A. retarded. Killers often kill again;
B. retarded killer is more to be feared
C. than a . . . normal killer.
D. There is also far less possibility of his
   ever becoming a useful citizen."

79. Lack of culpability because of
mental retardation

80. is simply not isolated at the sentencing
   stage

81. as a factor that determinatively bars a
   death sentence;

82. for individualized consideration at
   sentencing

83. is not designed to ensure that mentally
   retarded offenders

84. are not sentenced to death if they are
   not culpable

85. to the degree necessary to render
   execution a

86. proportionate response to their crimes.

87. When Johnny Penry is resentenced,

88. absent a change in Texas law,

89. there will be nothing to prevent the jury, acting lawfully,

90. from sentencing him to death once again --

91. even though it finds his culpability significantly reduced

92. by reason of mental retardation.

93. I fail to see how that result is constitutional,

94. in the face of the acknowledged Eighth Amendment

95. requirement of proportionality.

There is a second ground upon which I would conclude that the execution of mentally retarded offenders violates the Eighth Amendment:
1. killing mentally retarded offenders
2. does not measurably further the penal goals of either

A. retribution or
B. deterrence.
3, "The heart of the retribution rationale is
4. that a criminal sentence must be
5. directly related to the personal culpability
6. of the criminal offender."
7. Since mentally retarded offenders
8. as a class lack the culpability
9. that is a prerequisite
10. to the proportionate imposition of the death penalty,
11. it follows that execution
12. can never be the "just deserts" of a retarded offender,
13. blameworthiness by definition is not justly deserved.

Furthermore,
1. killing mentally retarded offenders
2. does not measurably contribute to the goal of deterrence.
3. It is highly unlikely
4. that the exclusion of the mentally retarded
5. from the class of those eligible to be sentenced to death
6. will lessen any deterrent effect the death penalty may have
7. for nonretarded potential offenders,
8. for they, of course, will under present

law
9. remain at risk of execution.
10. the very factors that make it
    disproportionate
11. and unjust to execute the mentally
    retarded
12. also make the death penalty of the most
    minimal deterrent effect
13. so far as retarded potential offenders
    are concerned.
14. "Intellectual impairments . . .
    A. in logical reasoning,
    B. strategic thinking,
    C. and foresight,"
    D. the lack of the intellectual and
    E. developmental predicates
    F. of an "ability to anticipate
       consequences," and
    G. "impairment in the ability to control
       impulsivity,"
    H. mean that the possibility of receiving
       the death penalty
    I. will not in the case of a mentally
       retarded person
    J. figure in some careful assessment of
       different courses of action.
    K. A person who has mental
       retardation
    L. often cannot independently generate
       in his mind
    M. a sufficient range of behaviors

N from which to select an action
O. appropriate to the situation
P. he or she faces (a particularly
    stressful situation)").
Q. In these circumstances,
R. the execution of mentally retarded
    individuals
S. is "nothing more than
T. the purposeless
U. and needless imposition of
V. pain and suffering,"
15, Because I believe that the Eighth
Amendment to the United States
Constitution stands in the way of a State
killing a mentally retarded
person for a crime for which, as a result of
his or her disability, he
or she is not fully culpable, I would reverse
the judgment of the
Court of Appeals in its entirety.

It is known that Traumatic Brain Injury
(TBI),
Attention Deficit Hyperactivity Disorder
(ADHD), and
Borderline Personality Disorder
(BPD)
have structural and functional
abnormalities of the frontal lobe and its
associated structures.

I rely on:
Structural and Functional Brain
Abnormalities
in Attention-Deficit/Hyperactivity Disorder
and
Obsessive-Compulsive Disorder: A
Comparative Meta-analysis
Luke J Norman, Christina Carlisi, Steve
Lukito, Heledd Hart, David Mataix-Cols,
Joaquim Radua, Katya Rubia
JAMA Psychiatry. 2016 Aug 1;73(8):815-825.
doi: 10.1001/jamapsychiatry.2016.0700.
PMID: 27276220 DOI:
10.1001/jamapsychiatry.2016.0700

And:

Depression, Anxiety, Anger, and
Behaviors, The Long View,
William R. Yee M.D., J.D.
Copyright Applied for March 21st, 2021

And:
Compared to controls,
1. the BPD group showed a reduced
GMV/Cth in prefrontal areas
2. but increased GMV in the limbic
structures
   A. amygdala and
   B. parahippocampal regions).

3. Prefrontal abnormalities correlated with
   A. higher baseline scores on impulsivity
      and
   B. general BPD severity.
4. Increased GMV in the parahippocampal
   area correlated with
   A. greater emotion dysregulation.
5. several baseline structural abnormalities
   correlated with
   A. worse response to psychotherapy.
6. Patients with BPD showed
   A. a reduced GMV in the prefrontal areas
   B. but a greater GMV in the limbic
      structures.
7. Several structural abnormalities
   A. middle and inferior prefrontal areas,
   B. anterior insula,
   C. or parahippocampal area
8. correlated with clinical severity and
9. could potentially be used as imaging
biological correlates
10. biomarkers to predict psychotherapy
    response.

I rely on:
Structural brain abnormalities in
borderline personality disorder
correlate with clinical severity and predict
psychotherapy response.
Brain Imaging and Behavior

Sampedro, F., Farrés, C.C.i., Soler, J. et al.
15, 2502–2512 (2021).
Accepted, 03 January 2021
Published, 26 February 2021
Issue DateOctober 2021
DOI https://doi.org/10.1007/s11682-021-00451-6

Borderline Personality Disorder
1. No class of psychoactive medication is consistently effective
2. No medications is FDA approved for Borderline Personality Disorder
3. Pharmacotherapy is not recommended For treatment of any core symptom of BPD
   A. marked emotional instability
   B. transient stress-related paranoid ideation
4. Functional magnetic resonance imaging studies have convincingly demonstrated
   A. pharmacotherapy does NOT change brain activity or connectivity,
   B. Psychotherapy
      i. ALTERS neural activities and
      ii. ALTERS connectivity of
   C. regions serving
      1. executive control
      2. emotion regulation
      3. dialectical behavior therapy and

D, psychodynamic therapies are effective.

I rely on:
Review of Borderline Personality Disorder
Falk Leichsenring, DSc; Nikolas Heim, MA, MSc3; Frank Leweke, MD1; et al
JAMA Published Online: February 28, 2023
Review

Judge Brennan's analysis of disabilities of mentally retarded applies equally to
1. people with dementia,
2. people with mental retardation and
3. people with brain damage due to
   A. Traumatic Brain Damage
     (TBI)
   B. Attention Deficit Hyperactivity
     (ADHD) Disorder
   C. Borderline Personality
     (BPD) Disorder

When people with TBI, ADHD, and BPD commit battery, assault, libel, and slander directed at the general population, the criminal justice system and the mental health system:
A. labeling them victims because of a
   history of
1. child abuse

2. PTSD
3. poverty
4. membership in a minority
B. Does not justify their criminal behavior
C. Does not justify releasing them into the community without supervision,
D. Does not serve the public welfare by releasing them into the community without supervision.

People diagnosed with
1. Oppositional Defiant Disorder,
2. Borderline Personality Disorder,
4. Mental Retardation,
4. Traumatic Brain Damage
Often present with concurrent diagnosis of:
1. Drug and Alcohol Use and Addiction,
2. Intermittent Explosive Disorder,
3. Adult Antisocial Behavior,
4. Antisocial Personality Disorder,
5. A lengthy criminal record.

There are no medications approved by the FDA for the treatment of Borderline Personality Disorder, Antisocial Personality Disorder or Criminal Behavior.

The Covid-19 Pandemic made a vivid display of flaws created by separating governmental agencies.

Governors arbitrarily sent Covid-19 patients to nursing homes, killing thousands of elderly who should have been quarantined from Covid-19 patients.

Jails and Prisons released thousands of criminals to avoid the costs of health care for Covid-19 patients resulting in a rise in murders and crimes by criminals that were convicted or not prosecuted.

Alaska has a small population, and its jails and prisons are combined and work closely with the state hospitals.

Alaska can become a leader in diagnosing and treatment criminals with mental illness.

The diagnosis and treatment of the mentally ill among criminals is complex. There are hundreds of variables in each case, more than the average health care worker can track with the current state of the art of Electronic Medical Records.

Alaska can use the latest technology of functional MRIs to
1. find structural and functional impairments of the brain and
2. track treatment with the aid of artificial intelligence to find effective interventions.

By combining the medical records of the state mental health system and the criminal justice system Alaska can start naming structural and functional abnormalizes of the criminally mentally ill and finding effective treatments for the structural and functional abnormalities of the criminally mentally ill.

The criminal justice system includes many minorities, many physically and mentally impaired, and many people who qualify for help under the banner of:
Diversity, Equity, and Inclusion.

Jails and prisons are the best starting point for addressing:
Diversity, Equity, and Inclusion.

Lessons learned in jails and prisons may be applied to the population at large.

For now, radicals, "influencers," and irrational people of all stripes compete for attention on social media, which distorts reality and rational resolution of social issues.

Inclusion of medical, political, academic, groups without narratives or agendas is ideal, and difficult.

I am here to do no harm and help if I can. Thank you for your time and attention.

Be kind and you can be my friend.

William R. Yee M.D., J.D.
Board Certified Psychiatrist.
Practicing Medicine and Psychiatry without interruption since 1972 in Michigan, Indiana, Kentucky, California, Texas, and now in Alaska at your service.

"Pre-Existing text," includes names of symptoms and medical illnesses, medications, people, corporations, law cases, statutes, text of statutes, the titles of articles and books, the content of articles and books cited, FDA Labels and FDA releases and images taken from the internet.

My copyright claim is a claim to the "original text," which is my personal experience as described in the text and my commentary on names of symptoms and medical illnesses, medications, people, corporations, law cases, statutes, text of statutes, the titles of articles and books, the content of articles and books cited, FDA Labels and FDA releases and images taken from the internet.